Crystal Healing & The Chakra System

Cara E. Moore, BSYA (Crys.) (Herb.)
FMANF, Yoga Teaching (Hatha Yoga)

ISBN: 0-9555394-3-9
ISBN-13: 9780955539435

DEDICATION

This book is dedicated to the healing art of Crystal Healing and the excellent training received by the British School of Yoga.

Table of Contents

ACKNOWLEDGMENTS

To the British School of Yoga for their excellent practitioner training. To my crystal suppliers for their high quality crystals and information. To the World Metaphysical Association for their accreditation for my crystal course.

1 HISTORY OF CRYSTAL HEALING

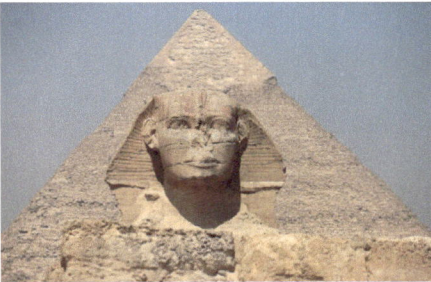

Ancient Egypt –Spynx

The Ebers papyrus (Egypt) states the medicinal uses of many different healing gem stones. Healing with crystals is also recorded in India's Ayurvedic records and in traditional Chinese medicine from around five thousand years ago.

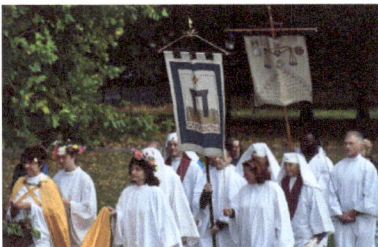

Druids –Autumn Equinox

Celtic tribes in Britain from as early as 2,000 B.C., were unified by a priesthood known as Druids. Druids are one of the earliest known peoples to have used crystals in divination.

"Our health, in shamanic terms, is the result of our empowerment, or lack of it. It is the result of our ability or inability to tap into the flowing light of creation." Celtic Shamism.com

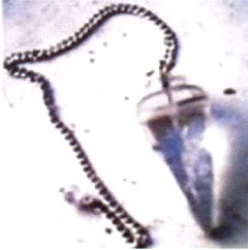

Clear Quartz Pendulum

Crystal Healing uses the Chakra System to "view" what is happening within the energy centers. By using a pendulum to test the sluggishness of a Chakra (by how freely the pendulum rotates) a "reading" can be taken and an appropriate crystal prescription can be made. Chapter 2 describes the Chakra Systems and what each chakra energy centre influences.

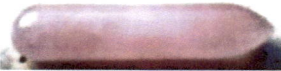

Rose Quartz Wand

A crystal wand is used to unblock Chakras and release negative energy, used pointed up and circle counter-clock wise to release negative energy and use pointed down and clock wise to put positive energy into the Etheric Body, which is the Auric copy of the physical body.

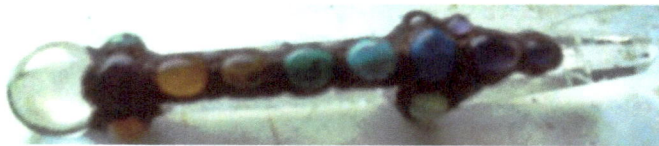

Chakra Clear Crystal Wand

This wand combines Chakra Crystals and Clear Quartz wand for use of the "master healer" clear quartz and extra boost of Chakra stones

2 SEVEN MAJOR CHAKRA SYSTEM

Crown Chakra – Clear Stones
Brow Chakra – Purple Stones
Throat Chakra – Blue Stones
Heart Chakra – Pink or Green Stones
Solar Plexus – Yellow Stones
Sacral Chakra – Orange Stones
Root Chakra – Red and Black Stones

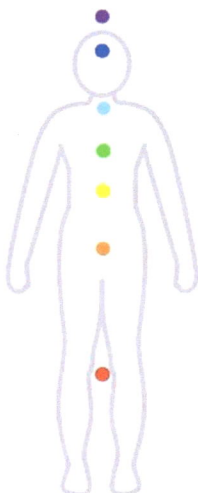

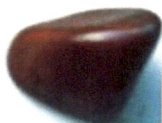

Red Jasper (Root Chakra)

ROOT CHAKRA

Located at the base of the spine. Colour is **red** (life energy) or **black** (signifying stability or grounding). Governs adrenal glands, it looks after our bones, teeth, nails, spinal column, anus, rectum, colon, prostate gland, blood and cell building, circulation. Concerns about security, money, survival, individuality.

Base Chakra gemstones are mostly red and black, including: Bloodstone, Red Coral, Garnet, Haematite, Brown Jasper, Red Jasper, Obsidian, Smoky Quartz, Ruby, Black Sapphire, Red Tiger Eye, Black Tourmaline.

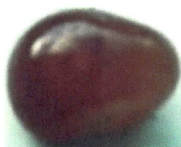

Carnelian (Sacral Chakra)

SACRAL CHAKRA

Located at about three inches below the navel. Colour is orange (representing creativity and wisdom). Sexual organs, pelvic area, kidneys, bladder, body fluids. The sacral chakra is associated with our relationships with others, our ability in giving and receiving, sexual /passionate love, and our creativity.

Sacral Chakra gemstones are mostly orange, including: Amber, Orange Calcite, Carnelian, Citrine, Orange Coral, Goldstone, Orange Jasper, Orange Sunstone, Tiger Eye and Topaz.

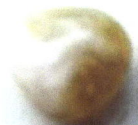

Citrine (Solar Plexus)

SOLAR PLEXUS CHAKRA

Located just below the ribs. Color is yellow (presenting thought and Self-determination). Pancreas, lower back, abdomen, digestive system, liver, spleen, gallbladder and nervous system. The Solar Plexus Chakra is our emotional centre. It aids in control of the "digestion of life", self-empowerment.

Solar Plexus Chakra gemstones are mostly yellow, including: Amber, Ametrine, Golden Beryl, Citrine, Yellow Jade, Yellow Jasper, Peridot, Smoky Quartz, Yellow Sapphire, Sunstone, Tiger Eye, Yellow Topaz and Yellow Tourmaline.

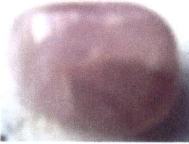

Rose Quartz (Heart Chakra)

HEART CHAKRA

Located at center of chest at the level of the heart. Color is **green** (healing and balance) or **pink** (unconditional love and compassion). Thymus gland, heart, upper back, lower lungs, blood, circulatory system and the skin. The heart chakra is about unconditional love, connection, acceptance, transformation and powerful healing. It is the centre of compassion, love, group consciousness and spirituality associated with a "oneness" with "all that is". Balances and bridges between the lower three chakras and the upper three chakras.

Heart Chakra gemstones are mostly green and pink, including: Amazonite, Green Aventurine, Green Calcite, Charoite, Chrysoprase, Emerald, Green Fluorite, Pink Fluorite, Jade, Green Jasper, Kunzite, Malachite, Peridot, Rhodochrosite, Pink Rhodonite, Rose Quartz, Green Sapphire, Pink Tourmaline, Green Tourmaline, Watermelon Tourmaline, Turquoise and Unakite.

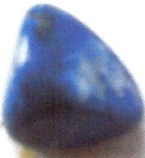

Lapis Lazuli (Throat Chakra)

THROAT CHAKRA

Located at the throat. Color is **blue** (Communication)

Thyroid gland, neck, throat and jaw, vocal chords, respiratory system, alimentary canal and arms. The throat chakra is our communication centre, enhances our ability to think and express ourselves verbally. Release of emotions, grieving, matters of the mind.

Throat Chakra gemstones are mostly blue, including: Amazonite, Amber, Angelite, Aquamarine, Azurite, Blue Lace Agate, Blue Calcite, Blue Chalcedony, Chrysocolla, Blue Fluorite, Lapis Lazuli, Malachite, Blue Sapphire, Sodalite, Blue Tiger Eye, Blue Topaz, Blue Tourmaline and Turquoise.

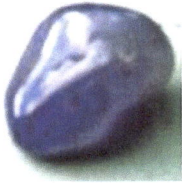

Amethyst (Brow Chakra)

THIRD EYE CHAKRA (BROW)

Located between and approximately one finger space above the brow. Color is **indigo** (spiritual search). Pituitary gland, face, left eye, ears, nose, sinuses, cerebellum (lower brain) and central nervous system. The third eye chakra is involved with our intuition, viewing our self-direction, higher consciousness, emotional and spiritual love centre.

Third Eye Chakra gemstones are mostlyindigo, including: Amethyst, Angelite, Azurite, Blue Calcite, Charoite, Purple Fluorite, Iolite, Lapis Lazuli, Lepidolite, Sapphire, Sodalite, Sugilite, Tanzanite and Turquoise.

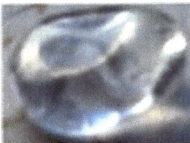

Clear Quartz (Crown Chakra)

CROWN CHAKRA

Located at the crown of the head. Color is **violet** (enlightenment) or White (purity, perfection and bliss). Pineal gland, it looks after our cerebrum (upper brain) and right eye. The crown chakra is the center of our connection to the Divine, the search for truth, self-awareness, material detachment.

Crown Chakra gemstones are mostly clear or violet, including: Amethyst, Ametrine, Angelite, Charoite, Diamond, Lepidolite, Clear Quartz, Sugilite and Tanzanite.

3 PREPARING STONES FOR USE

Cleansing

Gem stones are cleansed by using running water or Bach's remedy in spring water (especially useful at functions when used repeatedly).

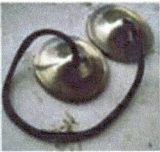

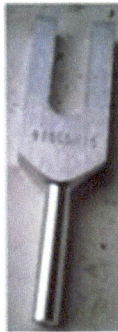

Tingsha Chimes   **Sounding Fork**

Tingsha chimes (sound) or a sounding fork can also be used to cleanse crystals as well as an area used for Healing.

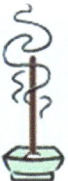   **Incense**

Passing crystals through incense such as sandalwood, frankincense, cedar or myrrh is also a traditional way of cleansing crystals and an area.

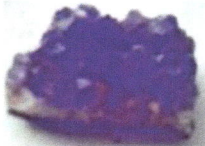

Amethyst Cluster

Charging

After crystals are cleansed they need to be charged. This can be done by placing them on crystal clusters.

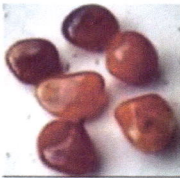

Carnelians

Charging can also take place by placing crystals with carnelian stones. Crystals can also be charged by placing in sunlight, cautions for Amethyst and Rose Quartz which can fade in sunlight.

Programming Dedication for Healing

Then they are then dedicated to healing through meditation before being used in Crystal Healing sessions.

4 PENDULUM USE

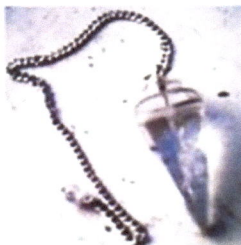

Clear Quartz Pendulum

Pendulums are an ancient tool used in healing that taps into the "higher consciousness" of the mind. Before using, establish "yes" and "no" direction. Pendulums are used in Crystal Healing sessions to see what "state" the Chakra energy centers are in and what blockages might exist. Pendulums can also be used when establishing which crystals or aromatherapy treatment to use. Pendulums serve a twofold purpose, as they are registering the energy levels they also repair at the same time and should be used several times during a healing session to monitor the effectiveness of the crystal treatments being used.

The British Society of Dowsers (www.britishdowsers.org.uk) publishes information on dowsing, provides workshops on the subject and has an online shop for the purchase of pendulums, dowsing equipment and books on related subjects. One such book is **The Definitive Wee Book on Dowsing** by Hamish Miller.

Sig Lonegren is a speaker and consultant on dowsing, labyrinths and sacred energy sites as well as an Honorary Life Vice President of the BSD and author of several books on dowsing and sacred energy sites.

Spiritual Dowsing by Sig Lonegren covers the subject of dowsing and its use in healing work. The **"A Little Book of Pendulum Magic"** by D. J. Conway is a compact but informative book on the history and uses of dowsing that includes charts for choosing crystals and aromatherapy treatments as well as stone meanings for pendulums.

Amethyst is noted as a healing pendulum.

Clear quartz pendulum as a protection crystal

Rose quartz is used to balance emotions, bringing love and healing.

5 CRYSTAL USES

Head and Eye: Azurite, Amethyst, Fluorite, Sugilite, Diamond

Ears, nose, throat and neck: Amazonite, Aquamarine, Blue lace agate, Celestite, Lapis lazuli, Kunzite, Preseli bluestone

Chest and lungs: Moss agate, Turquoise, Aventurine

Heart: Ruby, Aventurine, Emerald, Coral, Labradorite, Unakite

Digestion: Citrine, Tiger's Eye

Large intestines, kidneys, bladder: Obsidian, Peridot, Jade

Reproduction organs: Silver, Carnelian, Rhodocrosite, Moonstone, Selenite, Opal, Pearl

Circulation: Haematite, Bloodstone

Nervous System: Citrine, Silver, Gold, Sapphire, Rutilated quartz

Immune System: Turquoise, Aquamarine, Clear Quartz, Tourmaline, Chiastolite

Bones and muscles: Black Tourmaline, Lodestone, Spinel, Rutilated Quartz

Energy Boosting: Jet, Smoky Quartz, Tiger's eye, Garnet, Jasper, Amber, Gold

Uplifting: Petrified wood, Moldavite

Calming: Moonstone, Chrysoprase, Dumortierite

Stress reduction: Copper, Malachite, Haematite

Stabilizing Emotions: Sunstone, Kyanite, Dumortierite, Sapphire, Sodalite, Charoite, Rhodonite, Rose Quartz, Clear Quartz

6 IDENTIFYING STONES

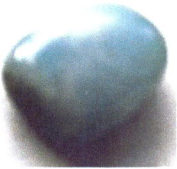

Amazonite – "Well being Stone", motivates, throat chakra. (See Amazonite Crystal Grid, Page 34) Sooths problems with ears, nose throat and nervous system, release blocked emotions.

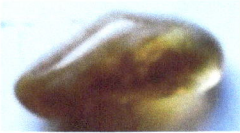

Amber – "Sun Power", solar plexus. Helps with nervous disorders, helps immune system, boosts energy.

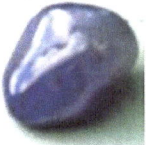

Amethyst – Healing Stone, spiritual, emotional balance, third eye Chakra. Aids meditation, sleep. (See Amethyst Crystal Grid, Page 32, 33)

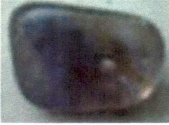

Ametrine - Combination of Amethyst and Citrine. Combats Depression, peace, tranquility, considered a powerful money stone.

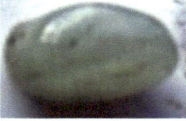

Aquamarine – Boosts immune system (thymus chakra, throat). Protection stone for sea travel. Encourages optimism, expression, inspiration.

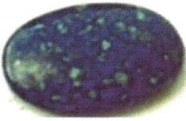

Azurite/Malachite –
Powerful combination for serious conditions. Azurite "clears out" deep-rooted emotions.

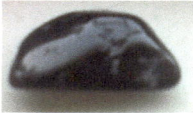

Black Tourmaline – Grounding, Protecting, Realigns, Root Chakra, soothes and settles bones and muscles. (See Black Tourmaline Grid, Page 35)

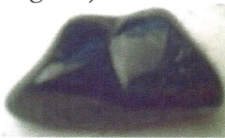

Bloodstone – Blood disorders, tumors. Energizes and balances heart and root Chakra. "Warrior stone". Has flecks of red, same composition as Green Jasper.

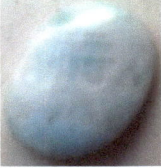

Blue Argonite – Pain relief, uplifting. Helps problem solving, useful for study for exams, tests. Releases stress, impatience.

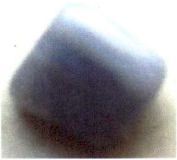

Blue Lace Agate – Fevers, Throat Chakra. Sooths emotions, anxiousness. Large tumble stone next to bed encourages restfulness.

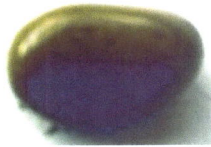

Carmel Agate – Earth stone, grounding. Protection and nurturing stone.

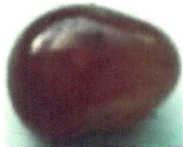

Carnelian – Sacral Chakra, pelvic area, bladder, body fluids. Protection stone, enhances creativity, repairs subtle bodies, releases stress, trauma. Boosts energy. (See Carnelian Crystal Grid Page 32)

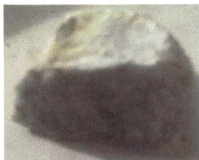

Celestite – Throat Chakra, Angel stone. Uplifting, Etheral. Opens mind to new ideas.

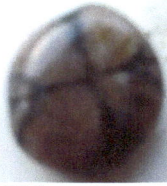

Chiastolite – Cross stone, protection. Given as a protection stone to people on pilgrimage. Used for fevers, balance immune system, rheumatism, strengthen nerves, increases lactation in nursing mothers. Helps combat depression, loneliness, isolation.

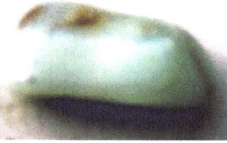

Chrysoprase- Detoxify and cleansing stone, promotes sound sleep, deep rest, calm and security. Increases creativity. Traditional good luck and success stone.

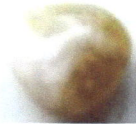

Citrine – Solar Plexus Chakra (Personal Self Power), Self Confidence, Warming. "sun energy". Known as "merchant's stone", kept in cash register to attract money.

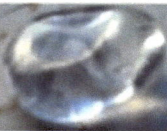

Clear Rock Quartz Balances all Chakras, known as the "master healer", Crown Chakra.

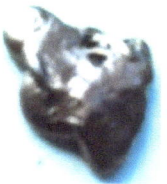

Copper – Reduces inflammation, used in bracelet form reduces pains of rheumatism and arthritis. Soothing.

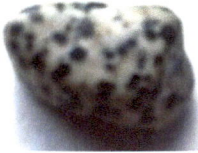

Dalmation Jasper – Nurturing, promotes calm, encourages courage and perseverance, good for stress and for pets experiencing trauma.

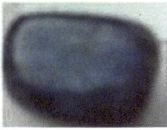

Dumortierite – Throat Chakra, patience, anxiety, stomach disorders caused by nervousness. Panic Attacks. calming.

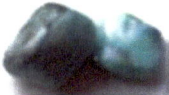

Emerald – Heart Chakra. Cleansing, Purifying, Calms, useful in meditation. Useful for healing Diabetes, Epilepsy. Encourages love, friendship, attachment. Caution: not to be worn continuously as may cause negative emotions.

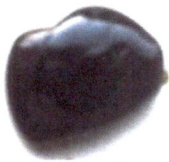

Garnet – Base Chakra. Speeds up healing process. Can be used with clear quartz healing wands for this purpose. Energizing, warming, good against cold, sluggishness and for improved circulation.

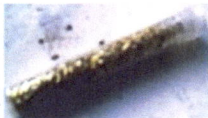

Gold – Strengthens immune system, stabilizes subtle electrical system. Boosts wealth, health, abundance. Place on areas needing healing. Useful as a gem essence. Place on heart chakra surrounded by clear quartz points to amplify infusion of life energy. Enhances self-confidence.

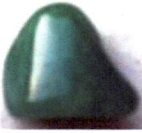

Green Aventurine – Balances heart Chakra. Spiritual growth, positive outlook, stabilizes emotions. Good for nerves, lungs.

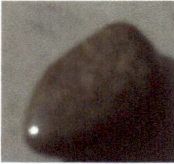

Green Jasper - Identical to Bloodstone without red flecks. Nurturing. Heart Chakra, Stability, Calming.

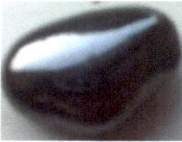

Haematite – Base Chakra, Protection stone, reduces inflammation, boosts self-esteem, grounding stone, Energizes.

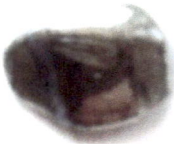

Healer's Gold - Gemstone of intellect and protection. Pyrite is also known as "healer's gold". Native American Indian's polished Pyrite and used it as a mirror.

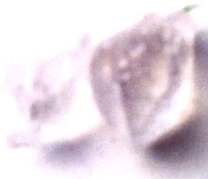

Herkimer Diamond – Powerful Detoxifier, wear over pancreas for Diabetes. Good for meditation. Found in Herkimer County, New

York state. Amplifier used by healers. Dispels darkness, balances energy flows.

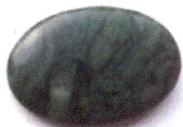

Jade – Longevity. Balances Heart Chakra, relaxes, promotes healing process. Sense of belonging. Considered lucky.

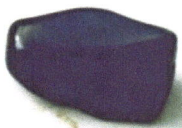

Jet – Calming, Grounding, lifts depression, balances when overburdened. Calms mind, Protection stone.

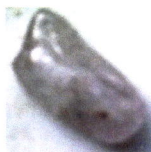

Kunzite – Brings resolution to a conflict, counters aggression, supports cardiovascular system, thyroid, enhances self-esteem. Combats negative thought patterns. Good for meditation. Trauma.

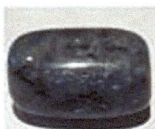

Kyanite – Throat Chakra. Calming, releases emotions, Useful for Meditation, Balances well being.

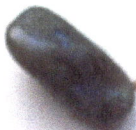

Labradorite – Protection stone, aura cleanser, focus, heart, inspiring, encouraging, solution solving.

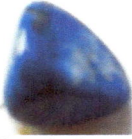

Lapis Lazuli – Throat Chakra, Truth, Balance and Justice. Protection stone, sends back harmful energies back to source in a healing way. Good for panic attacks, lungs, upper chest. Hearing complaints, use crystal grid of seven lapis, above head, beside each shoulder, by hands and feet, place five quartz near each ear, either side of solar plexus and between feet. Used in ancient Egypt. Afghanistan best source for Lapis.

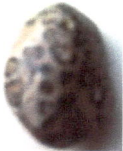

Leopard Skin Jasper - Balancing, nurturing, protection when travelling, doing Shamic work. "Stone of happiness and harmony".

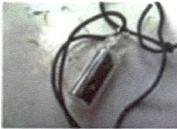

Lodestone – Pulls radiation, negativity from Aura when rotated through energy field, useful for t.v and computer radiation. Grounding. Turns adverse situations around. Aligns Chakras, subtle bodies. Realigns body to electromagnetic field of the planet.

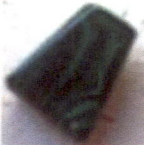

Malachite - Egyptian stone of "rebirth" Midwife stone. Relieves pain, helps recovery after exhaustion. Good in difficult situations, absorbs pollutants, corrects emotional imbalances, counteracts electromagnetic radiation, hold a malachite in each hand. Toxic, don't use in crystal essence, only use tumble stone for vibration, if broken, through away.

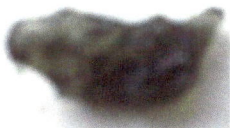

Moldavite – Amplifies properties of other stones, strengthen immune system, encourages innovation, true potential, transforming. Blends earthly and cosmic energies.

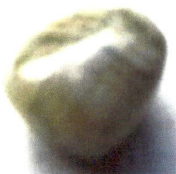

Moonstone – Emotional Balance, calming, balances body's blood and lymph systems, helps female issues, stress related indigestion, associated with fertility and growth.

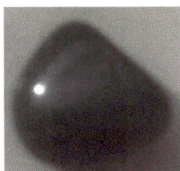

Moss Agate – Relaxing, connection to nature, releases emotions, optimism, sense of potential, congested area, circulation of blood, lymph. Useful for garden, plant one in each four corners of garden. Useful as room mood enhancer.

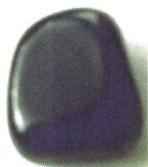

Obsidian - Revealing, cleansing transforming, polished used as a scrying tool. Rebalances digestive system. Grounding, protection stone. Brings hidden issues, emotions and traumas to the surface.

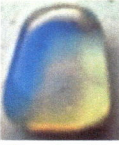

Opal – Eases flow of life energy through the subtle body. Helps stabilize mood swings. Delicate when exposed to air. Stabilizes emotions, increases sense of self-worth. Energizes Crown Chakra.

Pearl – Regulates glandular functions, assimilation of nutrients, balances emotions, increases tolerance, energizes sacral chakra, reduces, worry, anxiety, frustration, helps focus on who we are. To ease lower back pain, place pearl at sacral chakra, black tourmaline above head, below feet, lodestone at the base of neck. To release stress worry, or overcome addiction place pearl at solar plexus, clear quartz above head, smoky quartz or other grounding stone at feet.

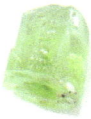

Peridot – Cleansing, Refreshing, Invigorating, removes toxins from body,combats negative train of thought. Strengthens personal identity, helps let go of past. Enhances natural healing processes, use with a grounding stone base of throat, one by heart, one near each kidney. Releases stress.

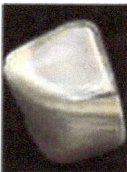

Petrified Wood – Earth stone, aids memory, stiffness in joints, restores energy to weakened parts of the body. Retains forest energy. Can see wood grain.

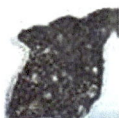

Preseli Blue – Stones used in inner circle of Stonehenge is a form of Dolerite found only in Preseli Mountains of Pembrokeshire, Wales. Grounding stone, stabilizes, relaxes and energizes, clarifies emotions, magical properties, doorway to other worlds, distant past.

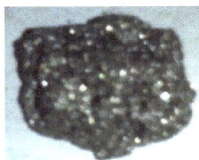

Pyrite – Cleansing, protects from pollutants, negative energy, grounding stone, detoxifying, good for anxiety, depression, frustration, uplifting, inspiring. Useful as a room mood enhancer.

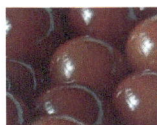

Red Coral – Root Chakra. Strengthens, protection, enhances life connection, empathic, heart, circulation and bones, balances emotions, boosts fertility.

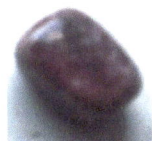

Rhodonite – Heart Chakra, good for Trauma, dispels negativity, anxiety, confusion. Useful for meditation.

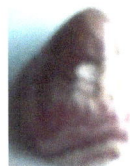

Rhodochrosite – Heart Chakra, good for Trauma, relieves anxiety, anger and pain, enhances self-worth, eases digestive and reproductive discomfort.

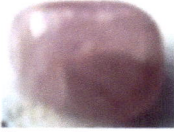

Rose Quartz – Heart Chakra, healing stone for burns, swelling, more gentle healing than Ruby. Good for relationships, called the "love stone".

Ruby - Root Chakra, powerful healer. Balances heart, physical and subtly. Confidence, security, self-esteem, warming. Grounding stone.

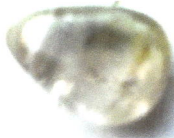

Rutilated Quartz – Helps to knit damaged tissue together, relax muscles, lightens mood, restoring, encouraging.

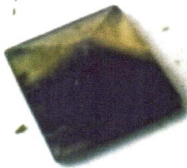

Purple Fluorite – Helps organization (place cluster or crystal in work area), anti-viral, inspiring, self confidence, Helps bone tissue, physical body.

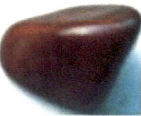

Red Jasper – Root Chakra, Grounding stone, nurturing, aids healing. Enthusiasm, drive, practical.

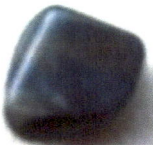

Sapphire – Throat Chakra, balances endocrine system, balances energies, calms, reduces tension, reduces fear, anxiety, stimulates mind, protection, encourages spiritual, attracts blessings, wisdom.

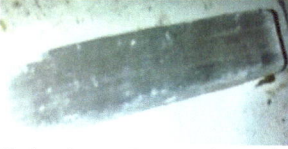

Selenite – Protection, clears darkness, negativity, cooling, removes long standing anger, resentment.

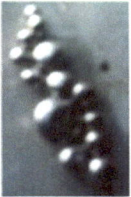

Silver – Prevents infections, eases flow, clears impurities, improves fertility, encourages intuition, eases difficulties with movement, and alleviates nervous twitches. Useful as a crystal gem essence.

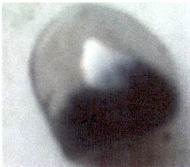

Silver Lace Agate – Nurturing, abundance, traditional protection stone, safety. Eases bad dreams, protects against energy drain.

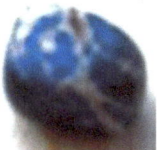

Sodalite - Throat chakra, cleanses lymphatic system, immune system builder, balances emotions, useful in meditation, encourages peace, contentment, relieves fear.

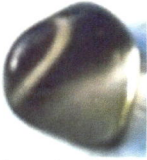

Smoky Quartz - Grounding stone, calming, useful in meditation, anti-radiation, stabilizes, concentrates energy.

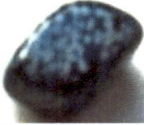

Snowflake Obsidian - Grounding stone, protection stone, brings traumas to surface, more gentle than black obsidian. Reveals, cleanses, transforms.

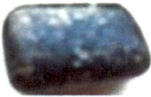

Spinel – Detoxifying, boosts energy flow, eases stiff muscles, transfers deep healing, inspiring, focus energy.

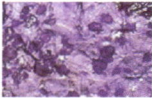

Sugilite – Reduces tension, gives practical focus for spiritual energies, stone for healers, nerves, helps coordination, learning.

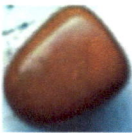

Sunstone – Uplifting. Happiness stone, self expression, artistic, warming, energizing, energy of sun, useful in meditation.

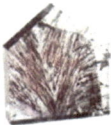

Super Seven- also known as Melody's Stone or Sacred 7, is a very spiritual stone. It is one of the few stones that retain their energy and clarity and never needs cleansing or energizing. Also, a piece of Super Seven retains the properties of all the stones in the combination of amethyst, smoky quartz, clear quartz, rutile, goethite, lepidochrosite and cacoxenite.

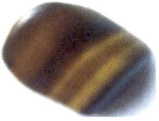

Tiger Eye – Solar Plexus Chakra. Protection (traditional stone against evil eye), useful for digestion, self-confidence, soothing, sociable interaction.

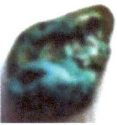

Turquoise – Healing stone, Throat Chakra, Protection stone, heart, thymus, neutralizes negativity, cooling, calming, strengthens aura.

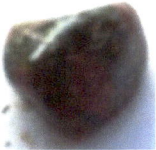

Unakite – Balances heart, circulation, soothes aches in pelvic area, enhances self worth, balances, creates perspective for problems, releases emotional blocks.

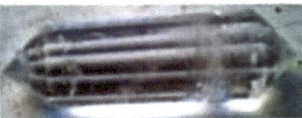

Vogel Cut Crystal – Cut specialized by Marcel Vogel a metaphysical scientist, useful in meditation, powerful healer, same resonance as holy water.

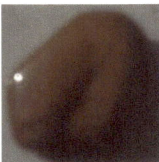

Yellow Jasper – Nurturing, Solar Plexus Chakra, "Protection Shaman stone". Useful for liver aliments.

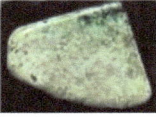

Zoisite – Powerful healer, detoxifier, stimulates healing, enhances creativity, individuality, helps fertility, helps recovery after illness.

7 HOW TO USE CRYSTAL GRIDS

Red or Black stones for Grounding Root Chakra (Garnet, Haematite)
Orange stones for Sacral Chakra (Carnelian)
Yellow stones for Solar Plexus (Citrine, Tiger Eye)
Green or Pink stones for Heart Chakra (Rose Quartz, Green Aventurine)
Blue stones for Throat Chakra (Blue Lace Agate, Sodalite)
Indigo stones for Third Eye(Purple Fluorite)
Purple or Clear stones for Crown Chakra (Amethyst, Clear Quartz)

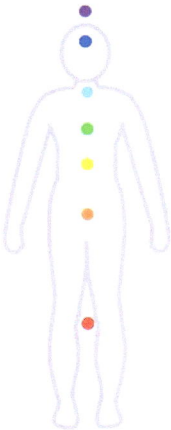

Carnelian Crystal Grid Layout

Carnelian Crystal Grid is an energy booster and healing grid, especially useful after an illness or when feeling rundown.

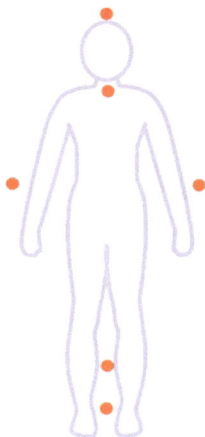

Amethyst Headache Layout

By focusing the amethyst clusters healing energy is directed to the head area.

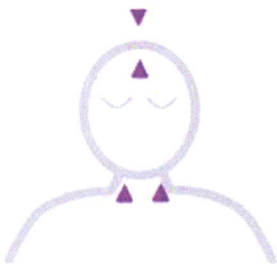

Moonstone Crystal Grid Layout

Moonstone Crystal Grid is a calming and relaxing nurturing grid useful when anxious and stressed.

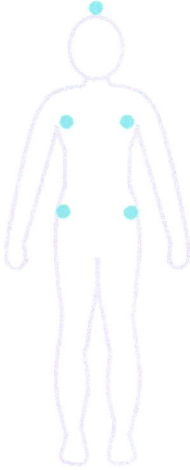

Amethyst Crystal Grid

Amethyst Crystal Grid is for intensive healing, especially useful to rebalance the aura and for chronic conditions, including stress.

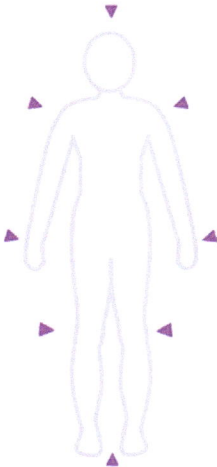

Amazonite Crystal Grid

Amazonite Crystal Grid is the "wellbeing" grid that soothes as well as motivates and gives focus to goals.

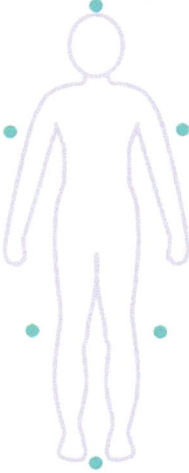

Solomon's Seal Crystal Grid

Solomon's Seal Crystal Grid uses clear quartz points and is useful for clearing negative energy from the Aura. First have the points pointing away from the body, then after 20 minutes, change to facing inward as shown to seal the Aura.

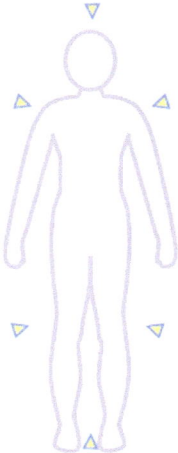

Black Tourmaline Crystal Grid

Black Tourmaline Crystal Grid is an intensive cleansing and protective grid used to clear longstanding negative energy and to repair tears in the auric field. Useful for grounding and stabilizing.

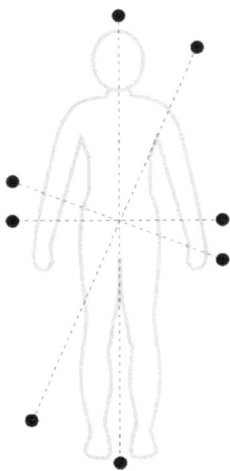

Therapy Room Setup

· Have clients take off their shoes and wear loose clothing.

· Pendulum is used to take energy readings and helps to pinpoint and clear areas of blockage.

· It is helpful to supplement these areas of blockage with relevant crystals or crystal grids to bolster recovery.

· Pendulum can be used to monitor correction of energy centers.

· Chakra Crystal Grid useful for Chakra Balance.

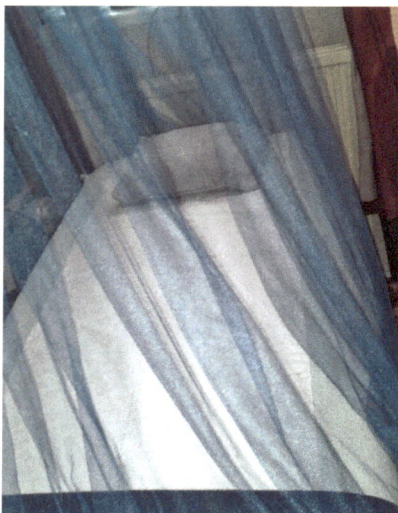

Beauty Therapy table, with cover, hygiene paper rolls, blankets, soothing music, aromatherapy, adjustable lighting.

8 MAKING CRYSTAL ESSENCES

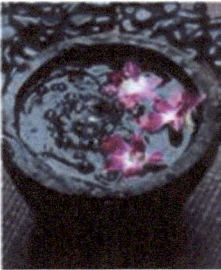

Making Crystal Gem Essences is an excellent way to use a crystals healing energy. Chakra Stones Crystal Gem Essences are helpful to boost recovery of energy blockages.

Gold and Jade are a useful tonic and balancer, Silver, helps combat infections, and Copper, to relieve inflammation are good essences to always have on hand. Black Tourmaline is a powerful protection and negative energy clearer. Purple Fluorite is an anti-viral and organizational booster.

Rose quartz is excellent for burns and swellings, wrinkles and Amethyst is a soothing pain reliever. Tiger Eye and Citrine are used for digestive complaints. Sodalite is useful for sore throats and communication issues. Garnet is used for circulation.

By soaking a crystal in spring water and placing it in the sun for two hours it transfers the crystal's energy to the water. (Use only quartz stones, don't use Malachite, as it is toxic). By putting crystal water in the fridge it can be kept for 2-3 days, to preserve as an essence for longer, brandy, vodka or apple cider can be used. (30%)

These essences can be drunk or used on pulse points or areas of concern, used as space clearance sprays or added to cosmetic products, such as hand cream.

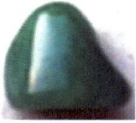

Averturine (Heart Chakra), Lungs, Heart, Nerves, Heart

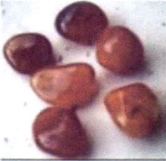

Carnelian Kidneys, (Sacral Chakra) Creativity, Pelvic Area, Sacral Chakra

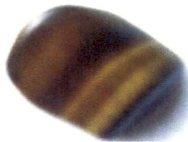

Tiger Eye (Solar Plexus) Self-confidence, digestion, Protection Stone

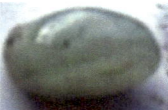

Aquamarine (Thymus Chakra) Immune system, Protection stone for sea travel, encourages, inspires.

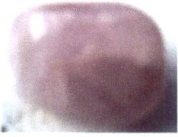

Rose Quartz (Heart Chakra) Burns, Swelling, Relationships, Gentle Healing

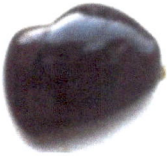

Garnet (Root Chakra) Circulation, Energy, Protection Stone

9 MEDITATIONS WITH CRYSTALS

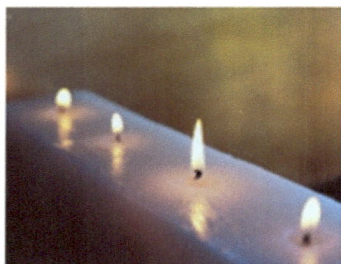

Candle Crystal Meditation

Kneel in front of crystal, facing north, light candle, meditate on light beings and light workers to be present with you, draw in white light, imagine it is filling your whole being, you will feel warmth and vitality passing through you, focus light in heart chakra, hold your hand over crystal and direct the light through your hand into the heart of the crystal. This is the dedication for love, freedom, truth and understanding.

Drawing white healing light into Crystal

Hold crystal in left hand, place right hand over crystal, draw in white light through crown chakra, feel it descending in your heart chakra, then visual energy being drawn in from deep within in the earth through the feet, this energy warms you until it settles in your solar plexus, now feel the white light in your heart, join the shape or a color take this symbol to your heart chakra, this will enable you to give your crystal unconditional love. Let the white light move from your heart through your hands and into the stone. You should feel the stone warming up as you do this, if not, repeat the process. You may dedicate the stone to truth, light and understanding.

Palm stones can be held during Crystal Healing Sessions and for Meditation.

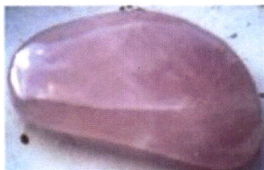

Rose Quartz – Heart Chakra, Burns, Swellings

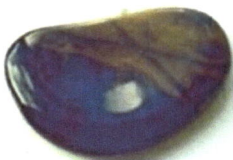

Tiger Eye –Palm stone Self-confidence, Digestive System, Solar Plexus Chakra

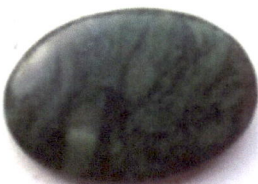

Jade Palm stone Good Balancer, Heart Chakra

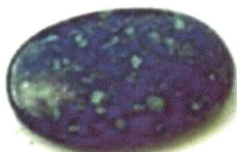

**Malachite/Azurite Palm stone
Good combination for deep healing**

INDEX

ABOUT THE AUTHOR

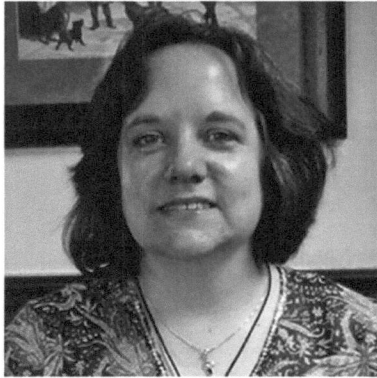

Cara E. Moore is a writer, poet and playwright who writes for Newspapers, Magazines and Internet sites, and whose play, The Healing won an honorable mention in the 1996 Writer's Digest Playwright Competition. She is the author of a collection of poetry <u>Horizon's Place And Time Meet</u>. She is also a Crystal Healing and Herbalism Practitioner and a Hatha Yoga Teacher, training at the British School of Yoga. She runs courses in Crystal Healing accredited by the World Metaphysical Association and runs workshops in Crystal Healing and has formulated a range of health and beauty products Crystal Essence ® available from Crystal Arts And Health.

www.ingramcontent.com/pod-product-compliance
Lightning Source LLC
Chambersburg PA
CBHW041227270326
41934CB00004B/187